YAKALOU MEDIA

Dating with Disabilities

100 Questions You Must Ask Yourself Before Dating a Disabled Person

First edition

This book was professionally typeset on Reedsy.
Find out more at reedsy.com

Contents

Disclaimer

This book is designed to provide information only. This information is provided and sold with the knowledge that the publisher and author do not offer any legal or other professional advice. In the case of a need for any such expertise, consult with the appropriate professional.

This book does not contain all the information available on the subject. This book has not been created to be specific to any individual's or organization's situation or needs. Every effort has been made to make this book as accurate as possible. However, there may be typographical and/or content errors. Therefore, this book should serve only as a general guide, not as the ultimate source of subject information.

This book contains information that might be dated and is intended only to educate and entertain. Regarding any loss or damage allegedly suffered or alleged to have occurred as a result of the information in this book, either directly or indirectly, the author and publisher shall have no liability or responsibility to any person or entity.

Introduction

Have you ever wondered what it takes to build a meaningful and loving relationship with someone who has a disability? This book, "Dating with Disabilities," is crafted to guide you through this very journey. It's not just a set of questions; it's a pathway to deeper understanding and empathy, crucial ingredients for any successful relationship, especially with individuals facing unique challenges.

Why are understanding and empathy so vital in relationships involving disabled individuals? Imagine walking a mile in their shoes and experiencing the world from their perspective. This book aims to open your eyes, broaden your mind, and prepare your heart for the beautifully rich yet often misunderstood world of dating someone with a disability.

In these pages, you'll find questions that may seem simple at first glance but delve deeply into your thoughts and feelings. These questions are designed to help you explore your own beliefs, confront any unconscious biases, and appreciate the complexities and joys of such a relationship. They will challenge you to think, reflect, and grow.

But why the questions? Because questions provoke thought. They lead us to answers we might never have considered. They encourage us to look within ourselves and to understand our own readiness to embark on this journey. From examining your communication skills to understanding daily practicalities, these questions cover a wide spectrum, ensuring you consider all aspects of such a relationship.

This book is more than just a guide; it's a conversation starter – with yourself and, eventually, with your partner. It's about laying a strong, compassionate foundation for a relationship that's built on more than just attraction – a relationship grounded in respect, understanding, and genuine love.

As you turn these pages, expect to embark on a journey of self-discovery and enlightenment. Each chapter builds upon the last, creating a comprehensive guide that prepares you for a relationship that is as rewarding as it is enlightening. Get ready to discover not just about the person you might date, but also about yourself. This is your first step towards building a relationship that celebrates love in all its diverse and wonderful forms.

The Rules to Get the Most Out of This Book

As you embark on this enlightening journey with "Dating with Disabilities," there are a few essential rules and a word of warning to keep in mind. These guidelines are designed not just to help you navigate through the book but also to ensure that you derive the most meaningful and authentic experience from it.

Rule 1: Honesty is Key

The first rule is simple yet profound: Be honest with yourself. As you go through the questions, it's crucial to answer them truthfully. This isn't about presenting yourself in the best light; it's about understanding your true feelings and perspectives. Only through honesty can you gain genuine insights and prepare yourself for a relationship that may be different from what you've known before.

Rule 2: Take Your Time

There's no rush. This book isn't something to breeze through. Reflect on each question, give yourself time to ponder your answers, and let the implications of these thoughts settle in your mind. The journey through these pages is as important as the destination.

Rule 3: Keep an Open Mind

Approach each question with an open mind. Preconceived notions or biases can cloud judgment and hinder growth. This book is a chance to challenge and expand your understanding, not just confirm what you already believe.

Rule 4: Embrace Discomfort

Some questions might make you uncomfortable. That's okay. Growth often happens outside our comfort zones. When you encounter a question that stirs unease, ask yourself why. The discomfort could be a sign of an area where you need more understanding or empathy.

Rule 5: Remember the Purpose

Keep in mind why you picked up this book. Whether it's to explore a potential relationship or to broaden your perspective, let this purpose guide your journey through the questions.

A Word of Warning

This book is not a checklist or a guarantee for a successful relationship. It's a tool to help you prepare and understand. Relationships, especially those involving disabilities, are complex and unique to each couple.

There is no one-size-fits-all approach. So, while this book can guide and inform, the actual journey of building and maintaining a relationship requires patience, love, and ongoing effort.

By following these rules and heeding this warning, you'll be able to make the most of this book. It's not just about reading; it's about engaging, reflecting, and growing.

The insights you gain here will be invaluable, not just in the context of dating someone with a disability, but in all aspects of understanding and embracing human diversity.

Chapter 1: Understanding Disabilities

This chapter delves into what disabilities are and how they can affect a person's life. When you're considering dating someone with a disability, it's crucial to have a clear understanding of what disabilities are. This knowledge helps in building empathy and appreciation for their experiences.

Disabilities come in many forms and can impact people in diverse ways. By learning about them, you're preparing yourself to connect more deeply and meaningfully with your partner.

Understanding Disabilities

1. Do I fully understand the nature of their disability?
2. Am I aware of the day-to-day challenges they might face due to their disability?
3. How does their disability affect their independence?
4. What can I learn about their specific disability?
5. Am I open to educating myself about disabilities in general?
6. How does this disability impact their mental and physical health?
7. Are there any misconceptions I might have about this disability?
8. What are the everyday needs of someone with this disabil-

ity?

9. How might their disability change over time?
10. Is there any specialized knowledge I need to acquire to understand their condition better?

Gaining knowledge about disabilities is the first step in appreciating and understanding your partner's world. This chapter aims to lay a solid foundation for that understanding, making you more empathetic and informed as you move forward in your relationship.

Chapter 2: Empathy and Sensitivity

Chapter 2 is all about empathy and sensitivity. When dating someone with a disability, being empathetic and sensitive to their needs and emotions is key.

This chapter guides you on how to be considerate and understanding, ensuring you provide the emotional support your partner needs. It's not just about understanding their disability, but also about understanding them as a person.

Empathy and Sensitivity

1. Am I sensitive to the feelings and needs of someone with a disability?
2. Can I empathize with the challenges they face?
3. How would I feel in their situation?
4. Am I prepared to be patient and understanding?
5. Do I recognize when to offer help and when to step back?
6. Can I handle situations where they might feel frustrated or limited by their disability?
7. Am I aware of the emotional support they might need?
8. How can I show that I respect their abilities and boundaries?
9. Am I comfortable talking about their disability with them?

10. Can I handle moments of discomfort or uncertainty empathetically?

Empathy and sensitivity are essential in any relationship, but they take on an added significance when your partner has a disability. This chapter helps you build these vital skills, ensuring you can be the supportive and understanding partner your significant other deserves.

Chapter 3: Communication Skills

Effective communication is the cornerstone of any healthy relationship, and this chapter focuses on enhancing your communication skills. It's especially important in relationships where a disability might affect the way you and your partner interact.

This chapter offers practical advice on improving communication, understanding non-verbal cues, and adapting to different communication styles.

Communication Skills

1. Do I know how to communicate effectively with someone who has a disability?
2. Am I comfortable asking questions about their disability when necessary?
3. Can I listen attentively and respectfully to understand their perspective?
4. Am I willing to adapt my communication style if needed?
5. How would I handle a situation where communication might be challenging due to their disability?
6. Am I prepared to learn new ways of communicating, like sign language, if necessary?

7. Can I express my own needs and feelings clearly and sensitively?
8. Do I avoid making assumptions about what they can or cannot do?
9. Am I open to discussing and resolving misunderstandings that may arise?
10. How can I ensure that our communication remains open and honest?

Mastering communication skills helps bridge gaps and strengthen your bond. This chapter equips you with the tools to communicate effectively with your partner, ensuring that you both feel heard and understood.

Chapter 4: Lifestyle Adjustments

Chapter 4 explores the changes you might need to make in your daily life when dating someone with a disability. These adjustments can range from small tweaks to significant alterations in your routine and living arrangements. Understanding and being ready for these changes is crucial for a harmonious relationship. This chapter helps you assess your flexibility and willingness to adapt, ensuring you can smoothly integrate your lives together.

Lifestyle Adjustments

1. Am I willing to make changes to my lifestyle to accommodate their needs?
2. Can I adapt to a different pace or style of living if required?
3. How would our dates and activities need to be adjusted to be inclusive for them?
4. Am I open to exploring new activities that are accessible for them?
5. Can I handle alterations in travel plans or living arrangements?
6. Am I prepared to spend time in environments that are designed for people with disabilities?
7. How would my daily routine change when dating someone

with a disability?

8. Am I ready to be flexible with plans, knowing that their needs might change unexpectedly?

9. Can I embrace a lifestyle that might include medical or therapeutic appointments?

10. Am I prepared for the financial implications of accommodating their disability?

Adapting to a new lifestyle is a significant part of dating someone with a disability. This chapter aims to prepare you for these changes, helping you embrace them with a positive attitude and an open heart, enhancing the quality of your relationship.

Chapter 5: Relationship Dynamics

In Chapter 5, we delve into the dynamics of a relationship when one partner is disabled. This includes understanding how a disability can affect emotional intimacy, physical connection, and social interactions.

It's important to recognize and navigate these dynamics sensitively and intelligently. This chapter provides insights and advice on maintaining a healthy, balanced, and fulfilling relationship.

Relationship Dynamics

1. How might their disability affect our emotional connection?
2. Can I maintain a balance between being a partner and a caregiver when needed?
3. Am I comfortable discussing topics related to their disability openly?
4. How will their disability impact our physical intimacy?
5. Can I handle the potential social dynamics and reactions from others regarding our relationship?
6. Am I prepared for the ways their disability might affect our future together?

7. How can we work together to build a strong and healthy relationship?
8. Are there specific accommodations or considerations we need to make for our relationship to thrive?
9. How can I ensure that our relationship remains equal and respectful?
10. Can I be a supportive partner during challenging times related to their disability?

Understanding and adapting to the unique dynamics of your relationship is key to its success. This chapter equips you with the knowledge and skills to navigate these dynamics effectively, ensuring a strong, loving, and resilient partnership.

Chapter 6: Support and Assistance

Chapter 6 focuses on the crucial aspects of support and assistance in a relationship with a disabled person. It's about understanding the fine line between helping and being overbearing.

This chapter guides you on how to offer support without infringing on your partner's independence. It's essential to learn the right ways to assist, ensuring that your help is empowering rather than disabling.

Support and Assistance

1. Do I know how to offer help without being overbearing?
2. Can I recognize when they need assistance and when they prefer to be independent?
3. Am I comfortable with the level of support they require?
4. How can I assist them in a way that respects their dignity?
5. Am I prepared to learn specific skills or techniques to provide appropriate support?
6. Can I handle the responsibilities that come with being a supportive partner?
7. How can I ensure that my assistance is empowering rather than disabling?
8. Am I willing to seek guidance or training if needed to

provide better support?

9. Can I respect their wishes when they decline help?
10. Am I prepared for the emotional aspects of providing support?

Offering the right kind of support and assistance is a delicate balance. This chapter helps you understand how to provide help in a way that respects your partner's autonomy and strengthens your bond, making your relationship more nurturing and respectful.

Chapter 7: Public Perception and Social Stigma

In Chapter 7, we address the societal aspects of dating someone with a disability. This includes handling public perceptions and overcoming social stigma. It's important to be prepared for various reactions from society and to support your partner through them.

This chapter provides strategies to deal with external opinions and misconceptions, fostering a strong and resilient relationship in the face of societal challenges.

Public Perception and Social Stigma

1. How will I handle others' misconceptions or judgments about our relationship?
2. Can I stand up against stigma or stereotypes related to dating someone with a disability?
3. Am I prepared to address inappropriate comments or questions from others?
4. How will I support my partner in public situations where they might face discrimination?
5. Can I be a positive advocate for disability awareness and inclusion?

6. Am I comfortable discussing our relationship with friends and family who might have biases?
7. How will I handle the attention our relationship might receive due to the disability?
8. Can I educate others about disabilities to help break down stigma?
9. Am I prepared to confront my own internalized biases or stereotypes?
10. How can I be a role model for respectful and inclusive behavior?

Dealing with public perception and social stigma can be challenging, but it's an important part of your journey. This chapter equips you with the tools to handle external pressures and maintain a healthy relationship, ensuring that you and your partner can thrive together despite societal challenges.

Chapter 8: Personal Growth and Learning

Chapter 8 is dedicated to exploring how dating someone with a disability can contribute to your personal growth and learning. It's about understanding how this unique relationship experience can broaden your perspective and enrich your life.

This chapter encourages you to reflect on the learning opportunities and how they can help you become a more compassionate, understanding, and well-rounded individual.

Personal Growth and Learning

1. What can I learn from this experience that will help me grow as a person?
2. How can this relationship enrich my understanding of diversity and inclusion?
3. Am I open to the life lessons that come with dating someone with a disability?
4. Can I use this experience to become more empathetic and understanding towards others?
5. How will this relationship challenge me and expand my worldview?
6. Am I willing to be vulnerable and learn from situations that

might be new or uncomfortable for me?

7. Can I embrace the unique perspectives and insights my partner brings due to their disability?

8. How can I use this experience to break down my own barriers and limitations?

9. Am I ready to grow and evolve through the challenges and joys of this relationship?

10. What personal strengths can I develop through this relationship?

Embracing the personal growth and learning that come with dating someone with a disability can be deeply rewarding.

This chapter helps you recognize and appreciate these opportunities, enhancing both your personal development and the quality of your relationship.

Chapter 9: Family and Friends' Reactions

In Chapter 9, we tackle the reactions you might encounter from your family and friends. Understanding and preparing for their responses, questions, and possible concerns are crucial.

This chapter offers advice on how to communicate effectively with your loved ones, ensuring they understand and respect your relationship.

Family and Friends' Reactions

1. How will I introduce my partner and their disability to my family and friends?
2. Can I handle potentially negative reactions from loved ones?
3. How will I support my partner if they face discomfort or rejection from my family or friends?
4. Am I prepared to educate my family and friends about disabilities?
5. Can I remain firm in my relationship choices despite others' opinions?
6. How will I handle questions or concerns from those close to me?

7. Can I be a bridge between my partner and my social circle?
8. Am I ready to stand by my partner if there is resistance or a lack of understanding from others?
9. How will I address any fears or misconceptions my family or friends might have?
10. Can I ensure that my partner feels welcomed and included in my social circles?

Navigating the reactions of family and friends is an important aspect of your relationship. This chapter provides guidance on handling these interactions with grace and confidence, helping to foster acceptance and support from your closest circle.

Chapter 10: Long-term Considerations

Introduction to Chapter 10: Long-term Considerations

The final chapter, Chapter 10, delves into the long-term considerations of dating someone with a disability. This includes discussing future plans, living arrangements, and potential caregiving scenarios. It's important to have open and honest conversations about the future. This chapter guides you through thinking about and discussing these topics, ensuring you and your partner are on the same page about your long-term goals and expectations.

Long-term Considerations

- Am I thinking about the long-term implications of dating someone with a disability?
- How do I envision our future together considering their disability?
- Am I prepared for potential changes in their health or abilities over time?
- How might their disability impact our plans for living arrangements, travel, or family?
- Can I commit to being with someone who may require ongoing care or support?

- Am I willing to discuss and plan for future caregiving responsibilities?
- How will we handle financial considerations related to their disability?
- Can I be adaptable and resilient in the face of unforeseen challenges related to their disability?
- Am I ready to engage in open and honest discussions about our future?
- How can we work together to create a fulfilling and sustainable life partnership?

Conclusion of Chapter 10

Considering the long-term aspects of your relationship is essential for building a strong, lasting partnership. This chapter helps you approach these topics thoughtfully and realistically, laying the groundwork for a fulfilling and enduring relationship. By addressing these considerations, you can build a solid foundation for your future together.

Conclusion

As we reach the end of "Dating with Disabilities," it's time to pause and reflect on the journey we've shared. Together, we've explored key insights about empathy, understanding, and the richness of human diversity. Each chapter was a step towards broadening our perspectives, not just about dating someone with a disability but about embracing the full spectrum of human connections.

Remember, this book is more than a collection of questions; it's a gateway to a journey of continuous learning and growth. Relationships, especially those involving a partner with a disability, are dynamic and evolving. They require patience, understanding, and a heart willing to learn and adapt. As you move forward, carry the lessons and insights from this book with you. Let them guide you in building a relationship that is not only loving but also deeply rooted in mutual respect and understanding.

Now, I would like to extend a heartfelt thank you for choosing this book. Your willingness to learn and grow is a powerful testament to the kind of partner you aspire to be. If this book has impacted you, I encourage you to share your experience by leaving a review. Your thoughts and reflections are not only valuable to me but also to other potential readers. Your review can guide them to this book, offering them the chance to embark on a similar journey of understanding and growth.

Your voice matters. By sharing your review, you play a vital role in spreading an important message—one of love, empathy, and acceptance. It's about creating a world where relationships flourish not just in spite of differences but because of them. Your review could be the beacon that guides someone to the understanding they need at a time when they need it most.

Thank you once again for your time, your open heart, and your commitment to understanding the beauty of diversity in relationships. May your journey ahead be filled with love, learning, and the joy of discovery.